MW00480349

ADRENAL RESET DIET JOURNAL
The Handy Companion Journal to Track Your Progress

ISBN-13:978-1505574067
ISBN-10:1505574064

Free Gift for You

To get your free copy of

"How to Stay Motivated
and Lose Weight"

visit

www.staymotivatedclub.com/adrenal

MEASURING YOUR SUCCESS

Weight Loss Chart

	Weight	Loss
Week 1		
Week 2		
Week 3		
Week 4		
Week 5		
Week 6		
Week 7		
Week 8		
Week 9		
Week 10		
Total Loss		

Body Measurements Chart

Measurement	Week 1	Week 3	Week 5	Week 7	Week 9	Inches Lost
Bust						
Chest						
Waist						
Hips						
Thigh						
Calves						
Upper arm						
Forearm						

BEFORE PICTURE

MY WEIGHT_____

WHAT I'M THINKING/HOW I FEEL: _____

_____

_____

_____

_____

_____

_____

DO NOT EAT THESE FOODS
Wheat
Dairy
Eggs
Sugar
(Additional Names for Sugar)

Buttered sugar	Diatase
Cane sugar	Maltose
Brown sugar	Malt sugar
Corn syrup	Mannitol
Cane juice	Florida crystals
Corn syrup solids	Molasses
Beet sugar	Sucrose
Confectioner's sugar	Sorghum syrup
Dehydrated cane juice	Sorbitol
Galactose	Yellow sugar
Agave nectar	Carob syrup
Demerara sugar	Treacle
Fruit juice concentrate	Lactose
Fructose	Panocha
Dehydrated cane juice	Raw sugar
Maltodextrin	Rice syrup

(Additional Names for Sugar, continued)

Diastatic malt	Castor sugar
HFCS (high fructose corn syrup)	Dextran
Glucose solids	Golden syrup
Barbados sugar	Fruit juice
Grape sugar	Glucose
Maple syrup	Date sugar
Honey	Ethyl maltol
Barley malt	Icing sugar
Refiner's syrup	Golden sugar
Sugar (granulated)	Turbinado sugar

WEEKLY MEAL PLANNER
Week of _____

	BREAKFAST	LUNCH	DINNER	SNACKS
MON				
TUE				
WED				
THU				
FRI				
SAT				
SUN				

🕐	MEAL TRACKING

DID I?

CARB CYCLE

YES   NO

☐   ☐

REPAIR MY CIRCADIAN RHYTHM	RAISE MY MENTAL CLARITY

DAY 2 – Date_____

🕐	MEAL TRACKING

DID I?

CARB CYCLE

YES   NO

☐   ☐

REPAIR MY CIRCADIAN RHYTHM

_____
_____
_____
_____

RAISE MY MENTAL CLARITY

_____
_____
_____
_____

DAY 3 – Date_____

🕐	MEAL TRACKING

DID I?

CARB CYCLE

YES   NO

☐   ☐

REPAIR MY CIRCADIAN RHYTHM

_____
_____
_____
_____

RAISE MY MENTAL CLARITY

_____
_____
_____
_____

🕐	MEAL TRACKING

DID I?

CARB CYCLE

YES   NO

☐   ☐

REPAIR MY CIRCADIAN RHYTHM

_____

_____

_____

RAISE MY MENTAL CLARITY

_____

_____

_____

🕐	MEAL TRACKING

DID I?

CARB CYCLE

YES   NO

☐   ☐

REPAIR MY CIRCADIAN RHYTHM

_____
_____
_____

RAISE MY MENTAL CLARITY

_____
_____
_____

DAY 6 – Date_____

🕐	MEAL TRACKING

DID I?

CARB CYCLE

YES   NO

☐   ☐

REPAIR MY CIRCADIAN RHYTHM

_____
_____
_____
_____

RAISE MY MENTAL CLARITY

_____
_____
_____
_____

DAY 7 – Date_____

🕐	MEAL TRACKING

DID I?

CARB CYCLE

YES NO

☐   ☐

REPAIR MY CIRCADIAN RHYTHM

_____
_____
_____
_____

RAISE MY MENTAL CLARITY

_____
_____
_____
_____

WEEKLY MEAL PLANNER
Week of _____

	BREAKFAST	LUNCH	DINNER	SNACKS
MON				
TUE				
WED				
THU				
FRI				
SAT				
SUN				

🕐	MEAL TRACKING

DID I?

CARB CYCLE
YES   NO
☐   ☐

REPAIR MY CIRCADIAN RHYTHM
_____
_____
_____

RAISE MY MENTAL CLARITY
_____
_____
_____

⏰	MEAL TRACKING

DID I?

CARB CYCLE

YES ☐   NO ☐

REPAIR MY CIRCADIAN RHYTHM

_____
_____
_____
_____

RAISE MY MENTAL CLARITY

_____
_____
_____
_____

🕐	MEAL TRACKING

DID I?

CARB CYCLE
YES   NO
☐   ☐

REPAIR MY CIRCADIAN RHYTHM
_____
_____
_____
_____

RAISE MY MENTAL CLARITY
_____
_____
_____
_____

🕐	MEAL TRACKING

DID I?

CARB CYCLE
YES   NO
☐   ☐

REPAIR MY CIRCADIAN RHYTHM
_____
_____
_____
_____

RAISE MY MENTAL CLARITY
_____
_____
_____
_____

🕐	MEAL TRACKING

DID I?

CARB CYCLE

YES   NO

☐   ☐

REPAIR MY CIRCADIAN RHYTHM

_____
_____
_____

RAISE MY MENTAL CLARITY

_____
_____
_____

🕐	**MEAL TRACKING**

DID I?

CARB CYCLE

YES NO

☐ ☐

REPAIR MY CIRCADIAN RHYTHM	**RAISE MY MENTAL CLARITY**
_____	_____
_____	_____
_____	_____
_____	_____

🕐	MEAL TRACKING

DID I?

CARB CYCLE

YES   NO

☐   ☐

REPAIR MY CIRCADIAN RHYTHM

_____
_____
_____
_____

RAISE MY MENTAL CLARITY

_____
_____
_____
_____

WEEKLY MEAL PLANNER
Week of _____

	BREAKFAST	LUNCH	DINNER	SNACKS
MON				
TUE				
WED				
THU				
FRI				
SAT				
SUN				

🕐	MEAL TRACKING

DID I?

CARB CYCLE

YES   NO

☐   ☐

REPAIR MY CIRCADIAN RHYTHM

_____
_____
_____

RAISE MY MENTAL CLARITY

_____
_____
_____

🕐	MEAL TRACKING

DID I?

CARB CYCLE

YES   NO

☐   ☐

REPAIR MY CIRCADIAN RHYTHM	**RAISE MY MENTAL CLARITY**
_____	_____
_____	_____
_____	_____

DAY 17 – Date_____

🕐	MEAL TRACKING

DID I?

CARB CYCLE

YES ☐ NO ☐

REPAIR MY CIRCADIAN RHYTHM
_____
_____
_____

RAISE MY MENTAL CLARITY
_____
_____
_____

🕐	MEAL TRACKING

DID I?

CARB CYCLE

YES   NO

☐   ☐

REPAIR MY CIRCADIAN RHYTHM

_____
_____
_____
_____

RAISE MY MENTAL CLARITY

_____
_____
_____
_____

DAY 19 – Date_____

🕐	MEAL TRACKING

DID I?

CARB CYCLE

YES ☐   NO ☐

REPAIR MY CIRCADIAN RHYTHM
_____
_____
_____

RAISE MY MENTAL CLARITY
_____
_____
_____

DAY 20 – Date_____

🕐	MEAL TRACKING

DID I?

CARB CYCLE

YES NO

☐ ☐

REPAIR MY CIRCADIAN RHYTHM

_____
_____
_____

RAISE MY MENTAL CLARITY

_____
_____
_____

29

🕐	MEAL TRACKING

DID I?

CARB CYCLE

YES   NO

☐   ☐

REPAIR MY CIRCADIAN RHYTHM	RAISE MY MENTAL CLARITY
_____	_____
_____	_____
_____	_____

WEEKLY MEAL PLANNER
Week of _____

	BREAKFAST	LUNCH	DINNER	SNACKS
MON				
TUE				
WED				
THU				
FRI				
SAT				
SUN				

🕐	MEAL TRACKING

DID I?

CARB CYCLE

YES   NO

☐   ☐

REPAIR MY CIRCADIAN RHYTHM	RAISE MY MENTAL CLARITY
_____	_____
_____	_____
_____	_____
_____	_____

🕐	MEAL TRACKING

DID I?

CARB CYCLE

YES   NO

☐   ☐

REPAIR MY CIRCADIAN RHYTHM

_____
_____
_____
_____

RAISE MY MENTAL CLARITY

_____
_____
_____
_____

DAY 24 – Date_____

🕐	MEAL TRACKING

DID I?

CARB CYCLE

YES   NO

☐   ☐

REPAIR MY CIRCADIAN RHYTHM	RAISE MY MENTAL CLARITY

🕐	MEAL TRACKING

DID I?

CARB CYCLE

YES   NO

☐   ☐

REPAIR MY CIRCADIAN RHYTHM

_____
_____
_____
_____

RAISE MY MENTAL CLARITY

_____
_____
_____
_____

🕐	MEAL TRACKING

DID I?

CARB CYCLE

YES   NO

☐   ☐

REPAIR MY CIRCADIAN RHYTHM	RAISE MY MENTAL CLARITY
_____	_____
_____	_____
_____	_____
_____	_____

🕐	MEAL TRACKING

DID I?

CARB CYCLE

YES   NO

☐   ☐

REPAIR MY CIRCADIAN RHYTHM	**RAISE MY MENTAL CLARITY**
_____	_____
_____	_____
_____	_____

🕐	MEAL TRACKING

DID I?

CARB CYCLE

YES   NO

☐   ☐

REPAIR MY CIRCADIAN RHYTHM

_____
_____
_____

RAISE MY MENTAL CLARITY

_____
_____
_____

WEEKLY MEAL PLANNER
Week of _____

	BREAKFAST	LUNCH	DINNER	SNACKS
MON				
TUE				
WED				
THU				
FRI				
SAT				
SUN				

🕐	MEAL TRACKING

DID I?

CARB CYCLE

YES   NO

☐   ☐

REPAIR MY CIRCADIAN RHYTHM

_____
_____
_____
_____

RAISE MY MENTAL CLARITY

_____
_____
_____

🕐	MEAL TRACKING

DID I?

CARB CYCLE

YES   NO

☐   ☐

REPAIR MY CIRCADIAN RHYTHM	RAISE MY MENTAL CLARITY
_____	_____
_____	_____
_____	_____
_____	_____

MIDWAY PICTURE

MY WEIGHT_____

WHAT I'M THINKING/HOW I FEEL: _____

_____

_____

_____

_____

_____

_____

🕐	MEAL TRACKING

DID I?

CARB CYCLE
YES   NO
☐   ☐

REPAIR MY CIRCADIAN RHYTHM
_____
_____
_____

RAISE MY MENTAL CLARITY
_____
_____
_____

🕐	MEAL TRACKING

DID I?

CARB CYCLE
YES	NO
☐	☐

REPAIR MY CIRCADIAN RHYTHM
_____
_____
_____

RAISE MY MENTAL CLARITY
_____
_____
_____

🕐	MEAL TRACKING

DID I?

CARB CYCLE
YES   NO
☐   ☐

REPAIR MY CIRCADIAN RHYTHM
_____
_____
_____
_____

RAISE MY MENTAL CLARITY
_____
_____
_____
_____

🕐	MEAL TRACKING

DID I?

CARB CYCLE

YES NO

☐ ☐

REPAIR MY CIRCADIAN RHYTHM	RAISE MY MENTAL CLARITY
_____	_____
_____	_____
_____	_____

🕐	MEAL TRACKING

DID I?

CARB CYCLE
YES   NO
☐   ☐

REPAIR MY CIRCADIAN RHYTHM
_____
_____
_____
_____

RAISE MY MENTAL CLARITY
_____
_____
_____
_____

This page intentionally left blank

WEEKLY MEAL PLANNER
Week of _____

	BREAKFAST	LUNCH	DINNER	SNACKS
MON				
TUE				
WED				
THU				
FRI				
SAT				
SUN				

DAY 36 – Date_____

🕐	MEAL TRACKING

DID I?

CARB CYCLE
YES   NO
☐   ☐

REPAIR MY CIRCADIAN RHYTHM
_____
_____
_____
_____

RAISE MY MENTAL CLARITY
_____
_____
_____
_____

🕐	MEAL TRACKING

DID I?

CARB CYCLE

YES　　NO

☐　　☐

REPAIR MY CIRCADIAN RHYTHM	RAISE MY MENTAL CLARITY
_____	_____
_____	_____
_____	_____
_____	_____

🕐	MEAL TRACKING

DID I?

CARB CYCLE

YES   NO

☐   ☐

REPAIR MY CIRCADIAN RHYTHM	RAISE MY MENTAL CLARITY
_____	_____
_____	_____
_____	_____
_____	_____

🕐	MEAL TRACKING

DID I?

CARB CYCLE
YES   NO
☐   ☐

REPAIR MY CIRCADIAN RHYTHM
_____
_____
_____

RAISE MY MENTAL CLARITY
_____
_____
_____

DAY 40 – Date_____

🕐	MEAL TRACKING

DID I?

CARB CYCLE
YES   NO
☐   ☐

REPAIR MY CIRCADIAN RHYTHM
_____
_____
_____
_____

RAISE MY MENTAL CLARITY
_____
_____
_____
_____

🕐	MEAL TRACKING

DID I?

CARB CYCLE

YES   NO

☐   ☐

REPAIR MY CIRCADIAN RHYTHM

_____

_____

_____

_____

RAISE MY MENTAL CLARITY

_____

_____

_____

_____

🕐	MEAL TRACKING

DID I?

CARB CYCLE
YES NO
☐ ☐

REPAIR MY CIRCADIAN RHYTHM
_____
_____
_____
_____

RAISE MY MENTAL CLARITY
_____
_____
_____
_____

WEEKLY MEAL PLANNER
Week of _____

	BREAKFAST	LUNCH	DINNER	SNACKS
MON				
TUE				
WED				
THU				
FRI				
SAT				
SUN				

DAY 43 – Date_____

🕐	MEAL TRACKING

DID I?

CARB CYCLE

YES   NO

☐   ☐

REPAIR MY CIRCADIAN RHYTHM	RAISE MY MENTAL CLARITY
_____	_____
_____	_____
_____	_____
_____	_____

🕐	MEAL TRACKING

DID I?

CARB CYCLE
YES   NO
☐   ☐

REPAIR MY CIRCADIAN RHYTHM
_____
_____
_____
_____

RAISE MY MENTAL CLARITY
_____
_____
_____
_____

🕐	MEAL TRACKING

DID I?

CARB CYCLE

YES   NO

☐   ☐

REPAIR MY CIRCADIAN RHYTHM	RAISE MY MENTAL CLARITY

🕐	**MEAL TRACKING**

DID I?

CARB CYCLE

YES   NO

☐   ☐

REPAIR MY CIRCADIAN RHYTHM	RAISE MY MENTAL CLARITY

DAY 47 – Date_____

🕐	MEAL TRACKING

DID I?

CARB CYCLE

YES   NO

☐   ☐

REPAIR MY CIRCADIAN RHYTHM

_____
_____
_____
_____

RAISE MY MENTAL CLARITY

_____
_____
_____
_____

DAY 48 – Date_____

🕐	MEAL TRACKING

DID I?

CARB CYCLE

YES   NO

☐   ☐

REPAIR MY CIRCADIAN RHYTHM
_____
_____
_____
_____

RAISE MY MENTAL CLARITY
_____
_____
_____
_____

🕐	MEAL TRACKING

DID I?

CARB CYCLE

YES   NO

☐   ☐

REPAIR MY CIRCADIAN RHYTHM	RAISE MY MENTAL CLARITY
_____	_____
_____	_____
_____	_____
_____	_____

WEEKLY MEAL PLANNER
Week of _____

	BREAKFAST	LUNCH	DINNER	SNACKS
MON				
TUE				
WED				
THU				
FRI				
SAT				
SUN				

🕐	MEAL TRACKING

DID I?

CARB CYCLE

YES   NO

☐   ☐

REPAIR MY CIRCADIAN RHYTHM	RAISE MY MENTAL CLARITY
_____	_____
_____	_____
_____	_____
_____	_____

🕐	**MEAL TRACKING**

DID I?

CARB CYCLE

YES   NO

☐   ☐

REPAIR MY CIRCADIAN RHYTHM

_____

_____

_____

RAISE MY MENTAL CLARITY

_____

_____

_____

🕐	MEAL TRACKING

DID I?

CARB CYCLE

YES   NO

☐   ☐

REPAIR MY CIRCADIAN RHYTHM	RAISE MY MENTAL CLARITY
_____	_____
_____	_____
_____	_____
_____	_____

🕐	MEAL TRACKING

DID I?

CARB CYCLE

YES   NO

☐   ☐

REPAIR MY CIRCADIAN RHYTHM

_____
_____
_____
_____

RAISE MY MENTAL CLARITY

_____
_____
_____
_____

🕐	MEAL TRACKING

DID I?

CARB CYCLE

YES   NO

☐   ☐

REPAIR MY CIRCADIAN RHYTHM	RAISE MY MENTAL CLARITY
_____	_____
_____	_____
_____	_____
_____	_____

🕐	MEAL TRACKING

DID I?

CARB CYCLE

YES   NO

☐   ☐

REPAIR MY CIRCADIAN RHYTHM

_____
_____
_____
_____

RAISE MY MENTAL CLARITY

_____
_____
_____
_____

DAY 56 – Date_____

⏰	MEAL TRACKING

DID I?

CARB CYCLE
YES   NO

☐   ☐

REPAIR MY CIRCADIAN RHYTHM

_____
_____
_____
_____

RAISE MY MENTAL CLARITY

_____
_____
_____
_____

WEEKLY MEAL PLANNER
Week of _____

	BREAKFAST	LUNCH	DINNER	SNACKS
MON				
TUE				
WED				
THU				
FRI				
SAT				
SUN				

🕐	MEAL TRACKING

DID I?

CARB CYCLE

YES   NO

☐   ☐

REPAIR MY CIRCADIAN RHYTHM

_____
_____
_____
_____

RAISE MY MENTAL CLARITY

_____
_____
_____
_____

🕐	MEAL TRACKING

DID I?

CARB CYCLE

YES   NO

☐   ☐

REPAIR MY CIRCADIAN RHYTHM

_____

_____

_____

RAISE MY MENTAL CLARITY

_____

_____

_____

🕐	MEAL TRACKING

DID I?

CARB CYCLE
YES   NO
☐   ☐

REPAIR MY CIRCADIAN RHYTHM
_____
_____
_____
_____

RAISE MY MENTAL CLARITY
_____
_____
_____
_____

🕐	MEAL TRACKING

DID I?

CARB CYCLE
YES   NO
☐ ☐

REPAIR MY CIRCADIAN RHYTHM	RAISE MY MENTAL CLARITY
_____	_____
_____	_____
_____	_____
_____	_____

AFTER PICTURE

MY WEIGHT_____

WHAT I'M THINKING/HOW I FEEL: _____

_____

_____

_____

_____

_____

_____

FAVORITE RECIPES

Recipe Name: _____
*Serves:*_____

Oven Temp_____Prep Time_____Cook Time _____

Ingredients:

_____   _____

_____   _____

_____   _____

_____   _____

Preparation Directions:

_____

_____

_____

_____

_____

Cooking Directions:

_____

_____

_____

_____

_____

Notes:

_____

_____

_____

_____

_____

FAVORITE RECIPES

Recipe Name: _____

*Serves:*_____

Oven Temp_____Prep Time_____Cook Time _____

Ingredients:

_____   _____

_____   _____

_____   _____

_____   _____

Preparation Directions:

_____

_____

_____

_____

_____

Cooking Directions:

_____

_____

_____

_____

_____

Notes:

_____

_____

_____

_____

_____

FAVORITE RECIPES

Recipe Name: _____
*Serves:*_____

Oven Temp_____Prep Time_____Cook Time _____

Ingredients:

_____   _____

_____   _____

_____   _____

_____   _____

Preparation Directions:

_____
_____
_____
_____
_____

Cooking Directions:

_____
_____
_____
_____
_____

Notes:

_____
_____
_____
_____
_____

FAVORITE RECIPES

Recipe Name: _____

*Serves:*_____

Oven Temp_____Prep Time_____Cook Time _____

Ingredients:

_____   _____

_____   _____

_____   _____

_____   _____

Preparation Directions:

_____
_____
_____
_____
_____

Cooking Directions:

_____
_____
_____
_____
_____

Notes:

_____
_____
_____
_____
_____

FAVORITE RECIPES

Recipe Name: _____

*Serves:*_____

Oven Temp_____Prep Time_____Cook Time _____

Ingredients:

_____   _____

_____   _____

_____   _____

_____   _____

Preparation Directions:

_____

_____

_____

_____

_____

Cooking Directions:

_____

_____

_____

_____

_____

Notes:

_____

_____

_____

_____

_____

FAVORITE RECIPES

Recipe Name: _____
*Serves:*_____

Oven Temp_____Prep Time_____Cook Time _____

Ingredients:

_____   _____

_____   _____

_____   _____

_____   _____

Preparation Directions:

_____
_____
_____
_____
_____

Cooking Directions:

_____
_____
_____
_____
_____

Notes:

_____
_____
_____
_____
_____

FAVORITE RECIPES

Recipe Name: _____
*Serves:*_____

Oven Temp_____Prep Time_____Cook Time _____

Ingredients:

_____   _____

_____   _____

_____   _____

_____   _____

Preparation Directions:

_____

_____

_____

_____

_____

Cooking Directions:

_____

_____

_____

_____

_____

Notes:

_____

_____

_____

_____

_____

FAVORITE RECIPES

Recipe Name: _____
Serves:_____

Oven Temp_____Prep Time_____Cook Time _____

Ingredients:

_____   _____

_____   _____

_____   _____

_____   _____

Preparation Directions:

_____

_____

_____

_____

_____

Cooking Directions:

_____

_____

_____

_____

_____

Notes:

_____

_____

_____

_____

_____

NOTES

NOTES

NOTES

NOTES

SHOPPING LIST

_____   _____

_____   _____

_____   _____

_____   _____

_____   _____

_____   _____

_____   _____

_____   _____

_____   _____

_____   _____

_____   _____

_____   _____

_____   _____

_____   _____

SHOPPING LIST

_____ _____

_____ _____

_____ _____

_____ _____

_____ _____

_____ _____

_____ _____

_____ _____

_____ _____

_____ _____

_____ _____

_____ _____

_____ _____

_____ _____

SHOPPING LIST

Made in the USA
Middletown, DE
09 May 2015